Light of Tai Chi

Denise Richard

ISBN-13:978-1539147596
ISBN-10:1539147592

DEDICATION

The Light of Tai Chi is of wholeness, a gift given by those who know that the power of heart and body are one. To the Grand Masters who have held this path and those who share the light I thank you. I dedicate this little book to Grand Masters Fu and Chen.

CONTENTS

ACKNOWLEDGMENTS

I acknowledge with joy those who come to this path to find health. I look to the power of practice and gratefully know the importance of honoring those who share this with heart. To those who have held my heart and taught me how to look to the light I offer this little book. May you walk the path of Tai Chi and know goodness.

1. LIGHT OF CHI

Pleasure in movement
as spirals create
emptiness in space
two with dragon

The pull of
movement was light
in opening with
strands of power

The strong shift
looks with something
unheard only so
energy will bound

Into clean view
of what will
now consist
this clear moment

2. ESSENCE OF MOVEMENT

The essence of Tai Chi is light throughout marked with usual movement of the body. In the Chinese tradition the use of gentle movement helps to make powerful the essence of chi so that the body can claim its full health and consciousness. This process is of value to the new student as the practice of movement deepens the experience of flow within.

Movement is consciousness expressed softly and gracefully, marked by the accentuation of a shift in weight with the sensitive engagement of hands and waist.

These together provide a healthy exercise that claim natural power in the body. The use of breath and the way of observation help to release stress, negativity and clear the mind. In all traditions of Tai Chi we see a common way of movement that respects the tradition of communal play and the building of a field of kindness.

The body is capable of expressing a movement that serves and in practice this means that the expression is of a making. For example, the process of learning hand movements teaches not only coordination and energetic awareness, but also respect for the balancing of the body and both hemispheres.

As the body ages there is a marked shift in connection with the earth. The practice of Tai Chi engages earthly power as support for the process of aging moves us to surrender and release. Mindfulness works and helps put pleasure into a simple walking exercise that claims good grounding.

Those who enjoy Tai Chi learn to observe a compassionate quality of flow in everyday life as the art teaches the student to move mindfully in accordance with a greater light.

3. DISTINCTIONS

The learning is from within as the practices of Tai Chi and Chi Kung help access a flow of consciousness and open energy pathways.

Though the practice of Chi Kung may sometimes be observed in special situations it is not Tai Chi practice. Chi Kung practices make use of multiple postures that inform and shift the energetic health in any level of awareness. The action of Chi Kung is subtle, stationary practice that supports awareness in consciousness; the play of Tai Chi is awareness through conscious whole body movement. Tai Chi focusses on the physical body and helps with coordination and breath. Both are of old and look to secure. The lineage sets the made intention of teaching ancient awareness in energetic health.

For the new student who chooses the way of Tai Chi there is first a sensitive learning of the mindfulness through slow movement. In the way of old, instruction began with very light practice such as the Tai Chi walk and single postures to gain health, awareness and grounding. With conscious breath and standard Tai Chi postures over a good period of time the student would learn the full practice.

This type of foundation clearly demonstrates a way of access for the light of Tai Chi is claimed through conscious repetitive movement without manipulation. The growth of the physical power is supported through the awareness that to heal and cleanses itself the flow of energy can only be observed. The joy of receiving a clean and clear practice through a great teacher is an incredible gift.

Tai Chi offers uniqueness in the honouring of tradition. Each tradition distinctively engages an understanding of growth through the value of each practice. The more involved the student becomes the greater the Tai Chi as the potent force of Chi grows through observation. The young student grows as each stage in life shifts the consciousness and value of practice. Here we come to respect the history of Tai Chi and the Masters who have claimed recognition for their persistence, power and presentation. The beauty of a culture rich in discipline and respect in awareness is of importance.

The knowing that there are different styles and different levels was brought to my awareness through the Grand Master of the Fu lineage where I was given a depth of knowledge and awareness of the roots and power of Tai Chi.

With his support I acquired knowledge of a way that had been perfected over many centuries as the way of Tai chi respects the building of and understanding of a greater light. Forms such as Bagua were born of observation of the relationship between the elements as in nature. Other forms may use multiple statements of a consciousness that mimics the animal kingdom as it holds itself in power. The movement itself is an energy that replicates and holds something of protection in the animal world. Therefore, a form that distinguishes movement and supports protection is considered of noble power.

Basics in practice are always of value since we need to continually renew our appreciation for simplicity and consciousness that help to secure form. In this a very small practice can help grow good health and profound awareness. This work was given through recognition as tradition speaks with light. The Fu style offers the shortest of forms and the most advanced of techniques, that when enjoyed mindfully support the light of Tai Chi.

When a teacher gives practice the student is able to reclaim a joy of being and the light is readily accessible. Knowing of this puts the student in awareness of the importance of the teacher, and asks for respect to be of sort. Together all this makes for a spiritual journey that is inclusive and securing.

4. LIGHT OF TAI CHI

Through the building of an awareness we learn that Tai Chi heals the body through stages. How the mind and body will claim this goodness is unique to each of us. For instance, in the beginning of our journey with the sensitive and gentle movement the mind may begin to show reticence when the flow of energy is maximised. Here the student begins to experience a lightness that will open and shift energetically the body and mind. For some this may feel challenging for the body may express fatigue or disinterest. All resistance is understood through a personal way of expression. This stage of growth may also be marked by a state of "no mind" or a feeling of "I can't". This may feel odd, since the work is so simple, yet this demonstrates how the body is learning to reclaim consciousness in which the mind will not play and of which the light of Tai Chi is in play.

For those who engage in this simple practice the honouring of the way is of acceptance. As the student becomes familiar and aware of how the body and mind demonstrate a personal sense of limitation with change, then light of Tai Chi is of choice.

The growth of conscious presence in the body through Tai Chi practice is of immense help for the student looking to reclaim health. The age of a student is of importance when the issue of health is of sort as a tiny practice can assist an elderly to claim good grounding and quiet health.

5. THE PRACTICE

The play of Tai Chi builds awareness in the body as it engages our internal world and creates union with the natural world. The practice is usually done outdoors to help the body calibrate with the environment through the seasons. The power of Tai Chi in practice involves the building of a protective energetic coating that supports the body to stay healthy and wise. The joy of having this level of health offers us the stability in making our life harmonious and sensitive.

The effortless experience of practicing in community offers a lightness that supports consciousness. When the light is secure and joy of sharing practice is given, the whole with vibrate in like. The way of Tai Chi is beauty and goodness for all.

UNDERSTANDING THE WAY

The sensitivity and awareness that we claim through Taoist practice ignites the creation of good grounding, clear heart and healthy relating. As we face discomforts and allow the way we chose to relate through acceptance.

As we accept the cause, effect and circumstances of a situation we can experience deep pain as it may ask that we recognize and respect the importance of other in the play of light. What is often not considered is a way of relating that does not misuse the power of relating. As we assess our reactions and how these affect others we pay gratitude for kind presence and holding of good association.

The power of the light of consciousness is given to the one who is present. This entails the honoring of that which is of good nature. To know a process that honors those given the power of Tai Chi is to claim an association of heart.

The power of the good earth field is where we allow ourselves to be. The way is to open to the field of light that is the awareness and path before us. Sometimes this is not easy since the way may look dangerous. Respect and acceptance for a greater consciousness reveals that regardless of what it seems the student is guided. This engages a field of awareness that moves the student through unusual circumstances. For those who learn this and know that there is no need for manipulation, an awareness of the play of light will continue to blossom and grow.

ABOUT THE AUTHOR

With three decades of practice and understanding of the ancient systems of Tai Chi and Chi Kung , Denise Richard is a qualified instructor. Her long standing dedication and support in offering the basic instruction is a service to you.

www.fiveblossomgatherings.com